AUTOIMMUNE HEPATITIS DIET COOKBOOK 2024

Nourish Your Body, Reclaim Your Health – Delicious Recipes and Lifestyle Strategies for Managing Autoimmune Hepatitis in 2024

FELIAK AKINS

Contents

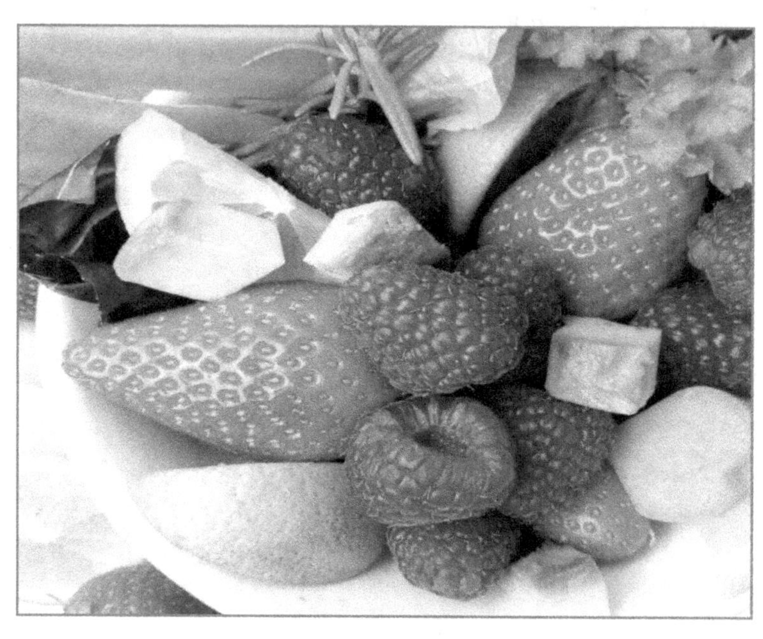

FRUITS

Introduction

Understanding Autoimmune Hepatitis

What is Autoimmune Hepatitis?

Welcome to the introductory section of "Autoimmune Hepatitis Diet Cookbook 2024." Before we embark on a culinary journey aimed at nourishing your body and managing autoimmune hepatitis through mindful eating, let's take a closer look at what this condition entails.

Understanding Autoimmune Hepatitis: A Brief Overview

Autoimmune Hepatitis (AIH) is a chronic liver disease that occurs when the body's immune system mistakenly attacks healthy liver cells, leading to inflammation and, over time, potential liver damage. Unlike other forms of hepatitis caused by viruses or lifestyle factors, AIH is classified as an autoimmune disorder.

Key Features of Autoimmune Hepatitis:

1. **Inflammation:** The immune system, designed to defend against harmful invaders, erroneously targets liver cells, causing persistent inflammation.

2. **Chronic Nature:** AIH is typically a long-term condition, demanding ongoing management and lifestyle adjustments.

3. **Varied Presentations:** The disease can manifest in various ways, ranging from mild symptoms to more severe forms that may progress to cirrhosis if left untreated.

4. **Unknown Cause:** The precise cause of autoimmune hepatitis remains unclear. Genetic predispositions, environmental factors, and infections may contribute to its development.

Diagnosis and Treatment:

AIH involves a combination of medical history assessments, blood tests, imaging studies, and sometimes liver biopsies. Once diagnosed, the primary goal is to manage symptoms and prevent further liver damage.

The Role of Diet in Autoimmune Hepatitis Management:

Diet plays a crucial role in managing autoimmune hepatitis, with certain foods and lifestyle choices having the potential to positively impact liver health. This cookbook aims to guide you through an Autoimmune Protocol (AIP) diet, emphasizing nutrient-dense, anti-inflammatory foods that support your overall well-being.

As we embark on this culinary adventure together, let's celebrate the power of intentional eating and lifestyle choices in promoting healing and restoring balance to your life. The recipes within these pages are crafted not only for flavor but also with a deep understanding of the intricate dance between food and well-being, offering you a roadmap to embrace health and vitality.

Impact on Liver Health

In the intricate symphony of our body's functions, the liver stands as a vital conductor, orchestrating processes essential for our well-being. As we delve into the pages of the "Autoimmune Hepatitis Diet Cookbook 2024," it becomes crucial to understand the profound impact autoimmune hepatitis can have on the health of this remarkable organ.

The Liver's Role in Health:

1. **Metabolism:** The liver serves as a metabolic powerhouse, regulating the conversion of nutrients into energy and maintaining glucose levels in the bloodstream.

2. **Detoxification:** It plays a central role in detoxifying the blood by breaking down and removing toxins from the body.

3. **Nutrient Storage:** The liver stores essential nutrients, including vitamins and minerals, ensuring a steady supply for the body's needs.

4. **Protein Synthesis:** Crucial proteins, such as those responsible for blood clotting, are produced by the liver.

Impact of Autoimmune Hepatitis on the Liver:

1. **Inflammation:** The immune system's misguided attacks lead to inflammation within the liver, hindering its normal functions.

2. **Impaired Detoxification:** Liver detoxification processes may be compromised, potentially allowing harmful substances to accumulate in the body.

3. **Cell Damage:** Continuous inflammation can result in damage to liver cells, impacting their ability to carry out essential functions.

4. **Risk of Cirrhosis:** In severe cases or when left untreated, autoimmune hepatitis can progress to cirrhosis, a condition where scar tissue replaces healthy liver tissue, affecting organ function.

The Interplay of Diet and Liver Health: Understanding the intricate dance between autoimmune hepatitis and liver health is crucial for effective management. The recipes and guidelines presented in this cookbook are tailored to not only tantalize your taste buds but also to nourish and support your liver on its journey to healing.

As we navigate the culinary landscape together, remember that each ingredient holds the potential to contribute not only to the flavor on your plate but also to the restoration of balance within your body. By embracing a diet rich in anti-inflammatory and nutrient-dense foods, you are not only savoring the delicious but also partaking in a healing ritual for your liver—a journey towards reclaiming vitality and well-being.

The Role of Diet in Managing Autoimmune Hepatitis

In the realm of autoimmune hepatitis, where the body's own defenses turn against the liver, the significance of a well-crafted diet cannot be overstated. As we embark on this culinary exploration within the "Autoimmune Hepatitis Diet Cookbook 2024," let's delve into the transformative role that diet plays in managing this complex and often challenging condition.

1. Nourishment as Medicine:

In the face of autoimmune hepatitis, every meal becomes an opportunity for healing. The foods we choose to consume can either exacerbate inflammation or serve as powerful allies in the body's quest for balance. This cookbook is not just a collection of recipes; it's a guide to utilizing the potent medicine found in your kitchen to support your liver's journey to recovery.

2. Anti-Inflammatory Embrace:

At the core of managing autoimmune hepatitis lies the concept of mitigating inflammation. The Autoimmune Protocol (AIP) diet, emphasized in this cookbook, strategically eliminates potential triggers and incorporates foods known for their anti-inflammatory properties. Through this approach, we aim to soothe the immune system's assault on the liver and create an environment conducive to healing.

3. Balancing Act:

Crafting meals that strike the right balance of nutrients is pivotal. Proteins, healthy fats, vitamins, and minerals all play essential roles in maintaining the liver's functionality and promoting overall well-being. The recipes provided are designed not only for their tantalizing flavors but also for their nutritional prowess, ensuring a harmonious balance in every bite.

4. Empowering through Choice:

Dietary choices empower us in our journey with autoimmune hepatitis. By understanding the impact of specific foods, we gain the ability to make informed decisions that positively influence our health. This cookbook serves as a roadmap, offering you the tools and knowledge to take charge of your diet and, consequently, your well-being.

5. Sustainable Lifestyle Shifts: Beyond individual meals, this cookbook advocates for sustainable lifestyle shifts. Mindful eating, stress reduction, and regular exercise are woven into the fabric of managing autoimmune hepatitis. These lifestyle elements complement the dietary recommendations, fostering a holistic approach to health.

As you flip through these pages and explore the delectable recipes that lie within, remember that each ingredient holds the potential to be a building block in your body's restoration. Together, let's celebrate the power of intentional and nourishing choices, transforming meals into a source of healing and resilience on your path to managing autoimmune hepatitis.

Each day is a step forward in your battle against Autoimmune Hepatitis. Embrace the progress, no matter how small, and let it fuel your determination for a brighter, healthier future

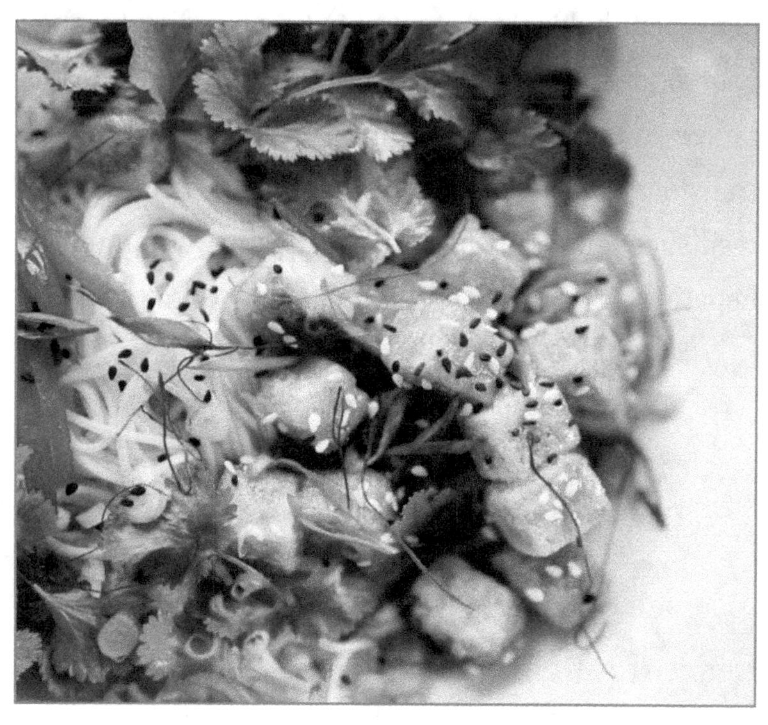

SALAD

Chapter 1: Foundations of AIP Diet

Introduction to the Autoimmune Protocol (AIP)

In the labyrinth of autoimmune hepatitis management, the Autoimmune Protocol (AIP) emerges as a guiding light—a comprehensive approach to harnessing the healing power of food. As we embark on Chapter 1 of the "Autoimmune Hepatitis Diet Cookbook 2024," let's unravel the principles and nuances of the AIP, a cornerstone in our journey toward nurturing well-being through intentional dietary choices.

1. Understanding AIP:

The Autoimmune Protocol is a therapeutic dietary framework designed to alleviate inflammation, manage autoimmune conditions, and support overall health. Initially derived from the Paleo diet, AIP takes a step further by eliminating additional potential triggers to the immune system.

2. Elimination Phase: Foods to Avoid:

AIP starts with a diligent elimination phase, steering clear of foods known to contribute to inflammation and autoimmune responses. Common culprits include gluten, processed foods, dairy, and refined sugars. By systematically excluding these triggers, we create a clean slate for the body, minimizing the chances of immune system flare-ups.

- *Gluten:* Found in wheat and related grains, gluten is known to trigger inflammatory responses, making its exclusion paramount in the AIP.

- *Processed Foods:* Laden with preservatives, additives, and artificial ingredients, processed foods can exacerbate inflammation, hence their exclusion.

- *Dairy:* Certain proteins in dairy may provoke immune reactions, making the removal of dairy products a crucial step in AIP.

- *Sugar and Artificial Sweeteners:* Refined sugars and artificial sweeteners may contribute to inflammation, prompting their elimination during the AIP phase.

3. Inclusion Phase: Nutrient-Dense Foods:

Following the elimination phase, AIP encourages the incorporation of nutrient-dense, whole foods that support healing and overall well-being. This includes an abundance of fruits, vegetables, lean proteins, healthy fats, and nuts and seeds.

- *Fruits and Vegetables:* Rich in vitamins, minerals, and antioxidants, these form the foundation of an anti-inflammatory diet.

- *Lean Proteins:* High-quality proteins aid in tissue repair and support the immune system without the potential triggers found in certain meats.

- *Healthy Fats:* Essential for cellular function and inflammation control, sources like avocados and olive oil are embraced in the AIP.

- *Nuts and Seeds:* Selected varieties rich in nutrients, while excluding those with high allergenic potential.

4. The Gradual Reintroduction Process:

AIP is not intended to be a lifelong restriction. Once a period of elimination has been followed and symptoms have improved, a gradual reintroduction of excluded foods is undertaken to identify individual tolerances and triggers.

5. Personalizing AIP:

Every individual's body responds uniquely. AIP serves as a foundational template, but personalization is key. Paying attention to your body's signals and working closely with healthcare professionals can help tailor the AIP to your specific needs.

As we embrace the principles of the Autoimmune Protocol, let this chapter serve as a comprehensive guide, offering both understanding and practical steps for implementing AIP into your daily culinary repertoire.

Chapter 2: Anti-Inflammatory Power Foods

Turmeric and Curcumin: A Golden Touch to Healing

In the vibrant palette of spices, turmeric stands out not only for its warm, golden hue but also for its remarkable healing properties. This chapter unfolds a culinary journey that embraces the potent duo of turmeric and curcumin—a golden touch to add not just flavor but also therapeutic benefits to your meals.

1. Turmeric Unveiled:

- **The Golden Root:** Turmeric, derived from the Curcuma longa plant, has been a staple in traditional medicine for centuries. Its vibrant color and earthy flavor make it a prized addition to various cuisines.

- **Curcumin's Star Power:** Curcumin, the active compound in turmeric, is responsible for many of its health benefits. Known for its anti-inflammatory and antioxidant properties, curcumin becomes a cornerstone in managing autoimmune hepatitis.

2. Benefits for Liver Health:

- **Anti-Inflammatory Action:** Turmeric's anti-inflammatory prowess can help reduce inflammation within the liver, a crucial aspect in managing autoimmune hepatitis.

- **Liver Detoxification Support:** Curcumin aids in promoting liver detoxification pathways, assisting the organ in clearing out toxins and maintaining optimal function.

- **Antioxidant Defense:** The potent antioxidants in curcumin contribute to neutralizing free radicals, offering protection to liver cells from oxidative stress.

3. Incorporating Turmeric into Recipes:

- **Golden Elixirs:** Turmeric lends itself seamlessly to various recipes. Golden milk, a beverage combining turmeric with warm milk, is a comforting way to enjoy its benefits.

- **Curry Creations:** Curries and stews become not just flavorful but also nutritious with the addition of turmeric. Explore diverse recipes that celebrate this spice's versatility.

4. Caution and Considerations:

- **Bioavailability Boosters:** Combining turmeric with black pepper enhances the absorption of curcumin, thanks to the presence of piperine.

- **Individual Sensitivities:** While generally safe, individual sensitivities can exist. It's advisable to start with moderate amounts and observe your body's response.

5. Recipe Inspirations:

- **Turmeric-infused Smoothie:** Blend turmeric with fruits, greens, and a splash of coconut milk for a refreshing and health-packed smoothie.

- **Turmeric-Spiced Quinoa Bowl:** Elevate a simple quinoa bowl with turmeric-infused vegetables, herbs, and a drizzle of olive oil.

6. Beyond the Plate:

- **Turmeric Supplements:** For those seeking a concentrated dose, turmeric supplements with standardized curcumin content are available. Consult with healthcare professionals before incorporating supplements.

As we venture into the heart of this chapter, let the warmth of turmeric and the potency of curcumin infuse your meals with not just flavor, but a golden touch of healing. Together, let's explore the culinary alchemy that makes turmeric a golden gem in the realm of autoimmune hepatitis management.

Ginger: Zestful Zing with Healing Grace

Let's turn our attention to ginger—a flavorful and aromatic root celebrated not only for its culinary prowess but also for its therapeutic benefits. Discover the zestful zing and healing grace that ginger brings to your autoimmune hepatitis management journey.

1. Ginger Unveiled:

- **Aromatic Allure:** Ginger, derived from the rhizome of the Zingiber officinale plant, boasts a distinctive spicy and citrusy flavor profile.

- **Gingerol's Magic Touch:** The bioactive compound responsible for ginger's unique taste, gingerol, holds anti-inflammatory and antioxidant properties, contributing to its health-promoting effects.

2. Anti-Inflammatory Properties:

- **Inflammation Taming:** Ginger's natural anti-inflammatory properties make it a valuable addition to a diet aimed at managing autoimmune hepatitis.

- **Cellular Defense:** Ginger's antioxidants help protect liver cells from oxidative stress, supporting overall liver health.

3. Adding Ginger to Daily Meals:

- **Ginger Tea Elixir:** A soothing cup of ginger tea can be a daily ritual, offering both comfort and anti-inflammatory benefits.

- **Stir-Fries and Curries:** Infuse stir-fries and curries with the vibrant flavors of fresh or ground ginger, elevating not just taste but also nutritional content.

4. Healing Ginger Recipes:

- **Ginger-Lemon Chicken Soup:** Create a comforting and nourishing chicken soup by incorporating fresh ginger and a hint of lemon for a revitalizing twist.

- **Ginger-Turmeric Smoothie:** Blend ginger with turmeric, pineapple, and yogurt for a refreshing and anti-inflammatory smoothie to kick start your day.

5. Ginger for Digestive Support:

- **Gut Soothing:** Ginger has been traditionally used to alleviate digestive discomfort, making it a valuable ally for those with autoimmune hepatitis.

- **Nausea Relief:** Ginger's anti-nausea properties can be particularly beneficial for individuals undergoing treatment or experiencing digestive challenges.

6. Caution and Considerations:

- **Moderation Matters:** While generally safe, it's advisable to consume ginger in moderation, especially for those prone to heartburn or with sensitivities.

- **Consulting Healthcare Professionals:** Individuals on specific medications should consult healthcare professionals before incorporating ginger into their routine.

As we immerse ourselves in the culinary landscape of autoimmune hepatitis management, let ginger be your flavorful companion—a zesty addition not only for its culinary charm but also for its potential to infuse your meals with healing grace. Together, let's embrace the therapeutic embrace of ginger, elevating both our dishes and our well-being.

Omega-3 Rich Fish: The Ocean's Gift for Liver Wellness

Now let's set sail into the ocean of nutritional benefits that omega-3 rich fish bring to the forefront of our autoimmune hepatitis management. Discover the aquatic treasures that not only tantalize the taste buds but also extend a helping hand to your liver's well-being.

1. The Omega-3 Advantage:

- **Essential Fatty Acids:** Omega-3 fatty acids, particularly EPA (eicosapentaenoic acid) and DHA (docosahexaenoic acid), are integral to supporting heart health, brain function, and notably, liver wellness.

- **Anti-Inflammatory Action:** The omega-3s found in fatty fish possess potent anti-inflammatory properties, making them a valuable asset in managing autoimmune hepatitis.

2. Importance of Omega-3 Fatty Acids:

- **Liver Support:** Omega-3s contribute to reducing inflammation within the liver, supporting its function and potentially mitigating the progression of autoimmune hepatitis.

- **Cell Membrane Integrity:** These fatty acids play a role in maintaining the integrity of liver cell membranes, enhancing their resilience against immune system attacks.

3. Fishy Goodness for Liver Health:

- **Fatty Fish Varieties:** Salmon, mackerel, sardines, and trout are among the oceanic delights rich in omega-3s, offering a delectable and health-promoting addition to your diet.

- **Grilled, Baked, or Broiled:** Explore various cooking methods to savor the rich flavors of omega-3 rich fish. Grilling, baking, or broiling are excellent choices that retain the nutritional benefits.

4. Incorporating Fish into Your Diet:

- **Regular Intake:** Aim for at least two servings of fatty fish per week to ensure a consistent supply of omega-3s.

- **Diversify Your Choices:** Experiment with different fish varieties to keep your meals exciting and to benefit from a spectrum of nutrients.

5. Fish Recipe Ideas:

- **Herb-Crusted Salmon:** Coat salmon fillets with a mix of herbs and bake for a flavorful and omega-3-rich dish.

- **Sardine Salad:** Combine sardines with fresh vegetables, herbs, and a light vinaigrette for a nutrient-packed salad.

6. Supplements Consideration:

- **Fish Oil Supplements:** For those with dietary restrictions or preferences, omega-3 supplements can provide a concentrated dose.

Consult healthcare professionals before incorporating supplements.

7. Caution and Considerations:

- **Mercury Levels:** While omega-3 rich fish are generally safe, be mindful of mercury content, especially for pregnant individuals. Choose low-mercury options such as salmon and sardines.

Dive into the depths of nutritional abundance with omega-3 rich fish, embracing not only the exquisite flavors of the sea but also the potential for enhanced liver health. Let this section inspire your culinary explorations, making omega-3 rich fish a delicious and nourishing cornerstone in your autoimmune hepatitis management journey.

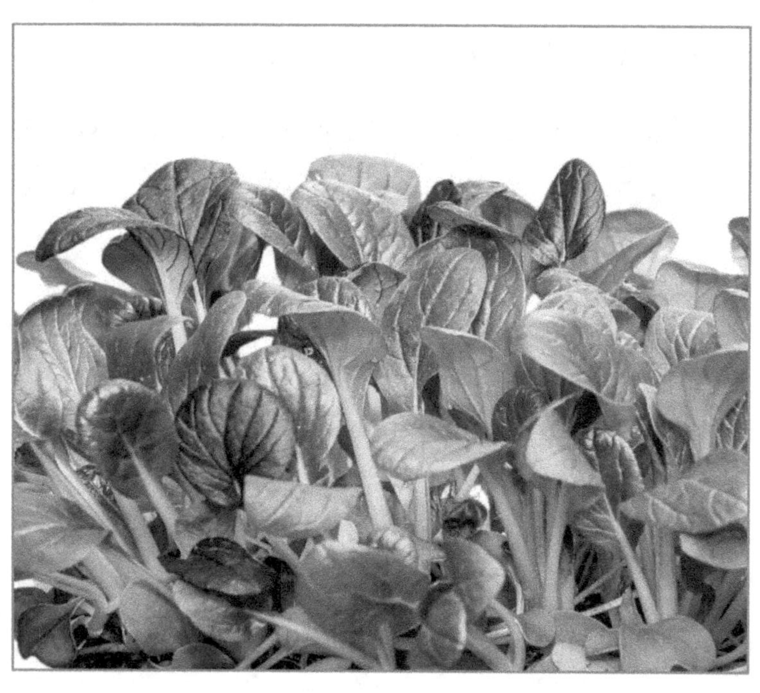

SPINACH

Chapter 3: Meal Planning and Recipes

Building AIP-Friendly Meals: Crafting Culinary Harmony for Healing

Welcome to Chapter 3 of the "Autoimmune Hepatitis Diet Cookbook 2024," where we embark on the art of building AIP-friendly meals – a symphony of flavors and nutrients carefully orchestrated to support your well-being. Let's explore the foundational principles of crafting meals that align with the Autoimmune Protocol (AIP), promoting healing and vitality.

1. A Foundation of Whole Foods:

- **Colorful Plate Palette:** Infuse your plate with an array of vibrant fruits and vegetables, providing essential vitamins, minerals, and antioxidants.

- **Lean Proteins:** Choose high-quality, lean proteins like poultry, fish, and grass-fed meats to support muscle health and overall well-being.

- **Healthy Fats:** Incorporate sources of healthy fats, such as avocados, olive oil, and coconut oil, to satiate and nourish your body.

2. Balancing Macronutrients:

- **Protein Power:** Ensure each meal includes an adequate protein source to support cellular repair and immune function.

- **Favorable Fats:** Opt for healthy fats that provide sustained energy and contribute to the absorption of fat-soluble vitamins.

- **Wholesome Carbohydrates:** Select carbohydrates from nutrient-dense sources like sweet potatoes and plantains, promoting digestive health and stable energy levels.

3. Sample Meal Plans:

- **Day-Breaking Nourishment:** Kickstart your day with a nutrient-packed smoothie bowl, blending fruits, greens, and a scoop of protein powder.

- **Power-Packed Lunch:** Enjoy a colorful salad with grilled chicken, mixed vegetables, and a drizzle of AIP-friendly dressing.

- **Dinner Delight:** Savor a baked salmon fillet with roasted sweet potatoes and a side of sautéed kale for a wholesome evening meal.

4. Mindful Portions and Frequency:

- **Portion Control:** Pay attention to portion sizes to avoid overeating and support digestive well-being.

- **Regular Meals:** Aim for regular, balanced meals throughout the day to maintain stable blood sugar levels and sustain energy.

5. Variety and Creativity:

- **Culinary Exploration:** Experiment with herbs, spices, and AIP-approved seasonings to elevate the flavors of your meals.

- **Recipe Adaptations:** Modify your favorite recipes to adhere to AIP principles, transforming them into delicious and health-promoting creations.

6. Preparing Ahead for Success:

- **Meal Prepping:** Streamline your AIP journey by preparing components of meals in advance, ensuring convenient and compliant options are readily available.

- **Batch Cooking:** Cook in batches and freeze portions for busy days, maintaining the convenience of wholesome AIP meals.

Crafting AIP-friendly meals is an opportunity to express creativity, relish delicious tastes, and fuel your body with intention. Let the ideas of balance, diversity, and mindfulness guide your culinary creations as you navigate this chapter, making every meal into a source of healing and well-being on your autoimmune hepatitis management path.

7-Day Autoimmune Hepatitis Diet Meal Plan

Day 1:

Breakfast:

- Turmeric and Ginger Infused Smoothie (Blend together coconut milk, pineapple, turmeric, ginger, and a handful of spinach.)

Lunch:

- Grilled Chicken Salad with Mixed Greens, Avocado, and AIP-Friendly Dressing.

Dinner:

- Baked Salmon with Lemon and Dill, Roasted Sweet Potatoes, and Steamed Broccoli.

Day 2:

Breakfast:

- AIP-Friendly Quinoa Porridge with Berries and a drizzle of Coconut Cream.

Lunch:

- Turkey and Vegetable Stir-Fry with AIP-Approved Sauce, served over Cauliflower Rice.

Dinner:

- Zucchini Noodles with Shrimp, Cherry Tomatoes, and Basil Pesto (AIP-friendly pesto made with olive oil, garlic, and basil).

Day 3:
Breakfast:

- Coconut Milk Chia Pudding topped with Mango and Kiwi.

Lunch:

- Tuna Salad Lettuce Wraps with Avocado and Cucumber Slices.

Dinner:

- Baked Chicken Thighs with Rosemary, Roasted Carrots, and Mashed Cauliflower.

Day 4:
Breakfast:

- Sweet Potato Hash with Ground Turkey, Spinach, and Turmeric.

Lunch:

- AIP-Friendly Butternut Squash Soup with a side of Mixed Berry Salad.

Dinner:

- Grilled Cod with Herbs, Sautéed Asparagus, and Quinoa.

Day 5:

Breakfast:

- AIP Smoothie Bowl with Pineapple, Banana, Coconut Milk, and AIP-Friendly Toppings (shredded coconut, sliced strawberries, and pumpkin seeds).

Lunch:

- Shredded Chicken Lettuce Wraps with Shredded Carrots and AIP-Friendly Tahini Dressing.

Dinner:

- AIP-Friendly Beef and Vegetable Stir-Fry served over Steamed Cauliflower Rice.

Day 6:

Breakfast:

- Green Plantain Pancakes with Fresh Berries and a drizzle of Honey (AIP-friendly honey substitute if needed).

Lunch:

- Turkey and Vegetable Skewers with AIP-Friendly Chimichurri Sauce, served with a side of Roasted Brussels Sprouts.

Dinner:

- Baked Trout with Lemon and Herbs, Sweet Potato Mash, and Steamed Green Beans.

Day 7:

Breakfast:

- AIP-Friendly Egg Muffins with Spinach, Tomato, and Turkey.

Lunch:

- AIP-Friendly Chicken and Vegetable Curry with Cauliflower Rice.

Dinner:

- Grilled Shrimp Skewers with Pineapple Salsa, Roasted Acorn Squash, and a side of Mixed Greens.

Remember to personalize portions according to your individual needs and consult with healthcare professionals for any specific dietary concerns. Enjoy this diverse and delicious 7-day Autoimmune Hepatitis Diet meal plan!

Autoimmune Hepatitis Diet Recipes

Breakfast Recipes

1. Turmeric and Berry Smoothie Bowl

Ingredients:

- 1 cup mixed berries (blueberries, strawberries, raspberries)

- 1 ripe banana, frozen

- 1/2 teaspoon turmeric powder

- 1 cup coconut milk (AIP-friendly)

- 1 tablespoon chia seeds

- 1 tablespoon shredded coconut (unsweetened)

Preparation:

1. In a blender, combine the mixed berries, frozen banana, turmeric powder, and coconut milk.

2. Blend until smooth and creamy.

3. Pour the smoothie into a bowl.

4. Sprinkle chia seeds and shredded coconut on top.

5. Enjoy immediately!

Nutritional Value:

- Calories: 350

- Protein: 5g

- Fiber: 12g

- Healthy Fats: 18g

- Carbohydrates: 40g

Cooking Time: 5 minutes

2. AIP Veggie Omelette

Ingredients:

- 2 large eggs (pasture-raised, if possible)

- 1/4 cup chopped bell peppers (mixed colors)

- 1/4 cup chopped zucchini

- 1 tablespoon fresh parsley, chopped

- Salt and pepper to taste

- 1 tablespoon coconut oil

Preparation:

1. In a bowl, beat the eggs and season with salt and pepper.

2. Heat coconut oil in a skillet over medium heat.

3. Add bell peppers and zucchini to the skillet and sauté until slightly softened.

4. Pour the beaten eggs over the vegetables and cook until the edges set.

5. Sprinkle with fresh parsley, fold the omelette, and cook until the eggs are fully cooked.

Nutritional Value:

- Calories: 250

- Protein: 14g

- Fiber: 2g

- Healthy Fats: 18g

- Carbohydrates: 6g

Cooking Time: 10 minutes

3. Sweet Potato and Spinach Hash

Ingredients:

- 1 medium sweet potato, grated

- 1 cup fresh spinach, chopped

- 1 tablespoon coconut oil

- 1/2 teaspoon turmeric powder

- Salt and pepper to taste

Preparation:

1. Heat coconut oil in a skillet over medium heat.

2. Add grated sweet potato and cook until it starts to brown.

3. Stir in chopped spinach and turmeric powder.

4. Continue cooking until the sweet potato is tender and the spinach is wilted.

5. Season with salt and pepper to taste.

Nutritional Value:

- Calories: 220

- Protein: 3g

- Fiber: 5g

- Healthy Fats: 10g

- Carbohydrates: 30g

Cooking Time: 15 minutes

4. Coconut Flour Pancakes

Ingredients:

- 1/4 cup coconut flour

- 2 large eggs

- 1/2 cup coconut milk (AIP-friendly)

- 1/2 teaspoon baking soda

- 1/4 teaspoon cinnamon

- 1 tablespoon coconut oil (for cooking)

Preparation:

1. In a bowl, whisk together coconut flour, eggs, coconut milk, baking soda, and cinnamon until smooth.

2. Heat coconut oil in a pan over medium heat.

3. Spoon small portions of the batter onto the pan to form pancakes.

4. Cook until bubbles appear on the surface, then flip and cook the other side.

Nutritional Value:

- Calories: 280

- Protein: 12g

- Fiber: 8g

- Healthy Fats: 15g

- Carbohydrates: 20g

Cooking Time: 10 minutes

5. AIP Banana Bread Muffins

Ingredients:

- 2 ripe bananas, mashed

- 3/4 cup coconut flour

- 3 large eggs

- 1/4 cup coconut oil, melted

- 1/2 teaspoon baking soda

- 1/2 teaspoon cinnamon

Preparation:

1. Preheat the oven to 350°F (180°C) and line a muffin tin with paper liners.

2. In a bowl, combine mashed bananas, coconut flour, eggs, melted coconut oil, baking soda, and cinnamon.

3. Mix until well combined.

4. Spoon the batter into the muffin tin, filling each cup about two-thirds full.

5. Bake for 20-25 minutes or until a toothpick inserted into the center comes out clean.

Nutritional Value:

- Calories: 180

- Protein: 6g

- Fiber: 6g

- Healthy Fats: 10g

- Carbohydrates: 20g

Cooking Time: 25 minutes

These recipes are not only delicious but also tailored to support the principles of the Autoimmune Hepatitis Diet. Adjust portion sizes as needed and consult with healthcare professionals for personalized advice. Enjoy your nourishing and flavorful breakfasts!

Lunch Recipes

1. Grilled Chicken Salad with AIP-Friendly Dressing

Ingredients:

- 4 oz grilled chicken breast, sliced

- 2 cups mixed greens (lettuce, arugula, spinach)

- 1/2 cucumber, sliced

- 1/2 avocado, diced

- A handful of cherry tomatoes, halved

- AIP-Friendly Dressing (olive oil, apple cider vinegar, Dijon mustard, salt, and pepper)

Preparation:

1. Grill the chicken breast until fully cooked, then slice.

2. In a large bowl, combine mixed greens, cucumber, avocado, and cherry tomatoes.

3. Add sliced grilled chicken on top.

4. In a small bowl, whisk together olive oil, apple cider vinegar, Dijon mustard, salt, and pepper to make the dressing.

5. Drizzle the dressing over the salad and toss gently.

Nutritional Value:

- Calories: 400

- Protein: 25g

- Fiber: 10g

- Healthy Fats: 25g

- Carbohydrates: 20g

Cooking Time: 15 minutes (for grilling chicken)

2. Turkey and Vegetable Stir-Fry with Cauliflower Rice

Ingredients:

- 1 cup ground turkey

- 1 cup broccoli florets

- 1/2 bell pepper, sliced

- 1/2 zucchini, sliced

- 1 tablespoon coconut oil

- 1 teaspoon ginger, grated

- 1 teaspoon turmeric powder

- Salt and pepper to taste

- Cauliflower Rice (store-bought or homemade)

Preparation:

1. In a pan, heat coconut oil over medium heat.

2. Add ground turkey and cook until browned.

3. Add broccoli, bell pepper, and zucchini to the pan.

4. Stir in grated ginger and turmeric powder.

5. Season with salt and pepper and continue to cook until vegetables are tender.

6. Serve over cauliflower rice.

Nutritional Value:

- Calories: 350

- Protein: 20g

- Fiber: 8g

- Healthy Fats: 15g

- Carbohydrates: 20g

Cooking Time: 20 minutes

3. AIP Butternut Squash Soup with Shredded Chicken

Ingredients:

- 2 cups butternut squash, peeled and diced

- 1 cup carrots, chopped

- 1 cup celery, chopped

- 1 onion, chopped

- 2 cloves garlic, minced

- 4 cups chicken broth (AIP-friendly)

- 1 cup shredded cooked chicken

- 1 teaspoon turmeric powder

- Salt and pepper to taste

- Fresh parsley for garnish

Preparation:

1. In a large pot, sauté onion and garlic until softened.

2. Add butternut squash, carrots, and celery to the pot.

3. Pour in chicken broth and bring to a boil.

4. Reduce heat and simmer until vegetables are tender.

5. Use an immersion blender to puree the soup until smooth.

6. Stir in shredded chicken and turmeric powder.

7. Season with salt and pepper.

8. Garnish with fresh parsley before serving.

Nutritional Value:

- Calories: 250

- Protein: 15g

- Fiber: 6g

- Healthy Fats: 10g

- Carbohydrates: 30g

Cooking Time: 40 minutes

4. Tuna Salad Lettuce Wraps with Avocado

Ingredients:

- 1 can tuna, drained

- 1/2 cup cucumber, diced

- 1/4 cup red onion, finely chopped

- 1/4 cup celery, finely chopped

- 1 tablespoon fresh dill, chopped

- 1 avocado, sliced

- Butter lettuce leaves for wrapping

- AIP-Friendly Lemon-Tahini Dressing

Preparation:

1. In a bowl, combine drained tuna, cucumber, red onion, celery, and chopped dill.

2. Spoon the tuna salad onto butter lettuce leaves.

3. Top with sliced avocado.

4. Drizzle with AIP-Friendly Lemon-Tahini Dressing.

Nutritional Value:

- Calories: 300

- Protein: 20g

- Fiber: 8g

- Healthy Fats: 18g

- Carbohydrates: 15g

Cooking Time: 10 minutes (if using canned tuna)

5. AIP-Friendly Chicken and Vegetable Curry with Cauliflower Rice

Ingredients:

- 1 lb boneless, skinless chicken thighs, diced

- 1 cup broccoli florets

- 1/2 cauliflower, riced

- 1/2 bell pepper, sliced

- 1/2 zucchini, sliced

- 1 can coconut milk (AIP-friendly)

- 2 tablespoons AIP-friendly curry powder

- 1 tablespoon coconut oil

- Salt and pepper to taste

- Fresh cilantro for garnish

Preparation:

1. In a pan, heat coconut oil over medium heat.

2. Add diced chicken and cook until browned.

3. Add broccoli, bell pepper, and zucchini to the pan.

4. Stir in AIP-friendly curry powder.

5. Pour in coconut milk and simmer until chicken is cooked through and vegetables are tender.

6. Season with salt and pepper.

7. Serve over cauliflower rice and garnish with fresh cilantro.

Nutritional Value:

- Calories: 400

- Protein: 25g

- Fiber: 10g

- Healthy Fats: 25g

- Carbohydrates: 20g

Cooking Time: 25 minutes

Dinner Recipes

1. Baked Salmon with Lemon and Dill

Ingredients:

- 2 salmon fillets (6 oz each)

- 1 tablespoon olive oil

- 1 tablespoon fresh dill, chopped

- 1 lemon, sliced

- Salt and pepper to taste

Preparation:

1. Preheat the oven to 400°F (200°C).

2. Place salmon fillets on a baking sheet.

3. Drizzle with olive oil and season with salt, pepper, and chopped dill.

4. Top with lemon slices.

5. Bake for 15-20 minutes or until the salmon flakes easily with a fork.

Nutritional Value:

- Calories: 350

- Protein: 30g

- Healthy Fats: 20g

- Omega-3 Fatty Acids: 1,500mg

- Cooking Time: 20 minutes

2. Zucchini Noodles with Shrimp and Pesto

Ingredients:

- 1 lb shrimp, peeled and deveined

- 4 medium zucchinis, spiralized

- 2 tablespoons AIP-friendly pesto (olive oil, garlic, basil)

- 1 tablespoon coconut oil

- Salt and pepper to taste

- Pine nuts for garnish

Preparation:

1. Heat coconut oil in a pan over medium heat.

2. Add shrimp and cook until pink and opaque.

3. Stir in spiralized zucchini and cook until just tender.

4. Toss with AIP-friendly pesto.

5. Season with salt and pepper.

6. Garnish with pine nuts before serving.

Nutritional Value:

- Calories: 300

- Protein: 25g

- Healthy Fats: 15g

- Fiber: 8g

- Cooking Time: 15 minutes

3. AIP-Friendly Beef and Vegetable Stir-Fry

Ingredients:

- 1 lb beef strips

- 2 cups broccoli florets

- 1 bell pepper, sliced

- 1 carrot, julienned

- 1 tablespoon coconut aminos

- 1 tablespoon coconut oil

- 1 teaspoon ginger, grated

- 1 teaspoon garlic, minced

- Salt and pepper to taste

- Fresh cilantro for garnish

Preparation:

1. In a wok or skillet, heat coconut oil over medium-high heat.

2. Add beef strips and cook until browned.

3. Stir in broccoli, bell pepper, and carrot.

4. Add grated ginger and minced garlic.

5. Drizzle with coconut aminos and stir-fry until vegetables are crisp-tender.

6. Season with salt and pepper.

7. Garnish with fresh cilantro before serving.

Nutritional Value:

- Calories: 400

- Protein: 30g

- Healthy Fats: 20g

- Fiber: 6g

- Cooking Time: 20 minutes

4. Herb-Crusted Chicken Thighs with Roasted Vegetables

Ingredients:

- 4 bone-in, skin-on chicken thighs

- 1 tablespoon olive oil

- 1 tablespoon fresh rosemary, chopped

- 1 tablespoon fresh thyme, chopped

- 1 teaspoon garlic powder

- 1 teaspoon onion powder

- 2 cups mixed vegetables (carrots, Brussels sprouts, cauliflower)

- Salt and pepper to taste

Preparation:

1. Preheat the oven to 375°F (190°C).

2. Rub chicken thighs with olive oil, chopped rosemary, thyme, garlic powder, and onion powder.

3. Place the chicken on a baking sheet.

4. Toss mixed vegetables with olive oil, salt, and pepper, and spread around the chicken.

5. Roast for 35-40 minutes or until the chicken is cooked through and vegetables are golden.

Nutritional Value:

- Calories: 450

- Protein: 35g

- Healthy Fats: 25g

- Fiber: 8g

- Cooking Time: 40 minutes

5. AIP-Friendly Turkey and Vegetable Soup

Ingredients:

- 1 lb ground turkey

- 4 cups bone broth (AIP-friendly)

- 2 carrots, sliced

- 2 celery stalks, chopped

- 1 sweet potato, peeled and diced

- 1 onion, chopped

- 2 cloves garlic, minced

- 1 teaspoon turmeric powder

- 1 teaspoon dried thyme

- Salt and pepper to taste

- Fresh parsley for garnish

Preparation:

1. In a large pot, brown ground turkey over medium heat.

2. Add carrots, celery, sweet potato, onion, and garlic to the pot.

3. Pour in bone broth and bring to a simmer.

4. Stir in turmeric powder and dried thyme.

5. Season with salt and pepper.

6. Simmer for 25-30 minutes or until vegetables are tender.

7. Garnish with fresh parsley before serving.

Nutritional Value:

- Calories: 350

- Protein: 25g

- Healthy Fats: 18g

- Fiber: 10g

- Cooking Time: 30 minutes

These dinner recipes are not only delicious but also tailored to support the principles of the Autoimmune Hepatitis Diet. Adjust portion sizes as needed and consult with healthcare professionals for personalized advice. Enjoy your nourishing and flavorful dinners!

Snacks Recipes

1. Avocado and Cucumber Slices with Lemon Zest

Ingredients:

- 1 avocado, sliced

- 1 cucumber, sliced

- Zest of 1 lemon

- Sea salt to taste

Preparation:

1. Arrange avocado and cucumber slices on a plate.

2. Sprinkle lemon zest over the slices.

3. Season with a pinch of sea salt.

4. Enjoy this refreshing and nutrient-dense snack.

Nutritional Value:

- Calories: 150

- Healthy Fats: 12g

- Fiber: 8g

- Vitamin C: 15mg

- Cooking Time: 5 minutes

2. AIP-Friendly Guacamole with Veggie Sticks

Ingredients:

- 2 ripe avocados

- 1/4 cup red onion, finely chopped

- 1/4 cup fresh cilantro, chopped

- 1 lime, juiced

- Carrot and cucumber sticks for dipping

Preparation:

1. In a bowl, mash avocados.

2. Stir in chopped red onion, cilantro, and lime juice.

3. Mix until well combined.

4. Serve with carrot and cucumber sticks for a crunchy and satisfying snack.

Nutritional Value:

- Calories: 200

- Healthy Fats: 16g

- Fiber: 10g

- Vitamin K: 30mcg

- Cooking Time: 10 minutes

3. Baked Sweet Potato Chips

Ingredients:

- 2 medium sweet potatoes, thinly sliced

- 2 tablespoons olive oil

- 1 teaspoon garlic powder

- 1 teaspoon paprika

- Sea salt to taste

Preparation:

1. Preheat the oven to 375°F (190°C).

2. Toss sweet potato slices with olive oil, garlic powder, paprika, and a pinch of sea salt.

3. Arrange the slices on a baking sheet in a single layer.

4. Bake for 15-20 minutes or until the edges are crispy.

5. Let cool before serving.

Nutritional Value:

- Calories: 180

- Healthy Fats: 8g

- Fiber: 6g

- Vitamin A: 15000IU

- Cooking Time: 20 minutes

4. AIP-Friendly Berry Smoothie

Ingredients:

- 1 cup mixed berries (blueberries, strawberries, raspberries)

- 1/2 cup coconut milk (AIP-friendly)

- 1 tablespoon chia seeds

- Ice cubes (optional)

Preparation:

1. In a blender, combine mixed berries, coconut milk, and chia seeds.

2. Blend until smooth.

3. Add ice cubes if desired and blend again.

4. Pour into a glass and enjoy this antioxidant-rich smoothie.

Nutritional Value:

- Calories: 150

- Protein: 3g

- Healthy Fats: 8g

- Fiber: 8g

- Cooking Time: 5 minutes

5. AIP-Friendly Trail Mix

Ingredients:

- 1/2 cup coconut flakes (unsweetened)

- 1/2 cup pumpkin seeds

- 1/2 cup dried cranberries (sweetened with apple juice)

- 1/4 cup sliced almonds

- 1/4 cup dried apricots, chopped

Preparation:

1. In a bowl, combine coconut flakes, pumpkin seeds, dried cranberries, sliced almonds, and chopped dried apricots.

2. Mix well.

3. Portion into small snack-sized bags for convenient, on-the-go munching.

Nutritional Value:

- Calories: 250

- Protein: 8g

- Healthy Fats: 15g

- Fiber: 6g

- Cooking Time: 5 minutes

These snack recipes are designed to align with the principles of the Autoimmune Hepatitis Diet. Adjust portion sizes as needed and consult with healthcare professionals for personalized advice. Enjoy these wholesome and satisfying snacks on your journey to better health!

Desserts Recipes

1. AIP-Friendly Berry Sorbet

Ingredients:

- 2 cups mixed berries (blueberries, strawberries, raspberries)

- 1 tablespoon honey (AIP-friendly)

- 1 tablespoon fresh mint leaves

- 1 tablespoon coconut water

Preparation:

1. In a blender, combine mixed berries, honey, fresh mint leaves, and coconut water.

2. Blend until smooth.

3. Pour the mixture into a shallow dish and freeze for at least 4 hours.

4. Before serving, let it sit at room temperature for a few minutes to soften.

5. Scoop into bowls and garnish with additional mint leaves.

Nutritional Value:

- Calories: 120

- Fiber: 8g

- Vitamin C: 30mg

- Antioxidants: High

- Cooking Time: 10 minutes + freezing time

2. AIP-Friendly Apple Cinnamon Baked Pears

Ingredients:

- 2 ripe but firm pears, halved and cored

- 1 tablespoon coconut oil, melted

- 1 teaspoon cinnamon

- 1 tablespoon shredded coconut (unsweetened)

- 1 tablespoon chopped walnuts

Preparation:

1. Preheat the oven to 375°F (190°C).

2. Place pear halves in a baking dish.

3. Drizzle with melted coconut oil and sprinkle with cinnamon.

4. Bake for 20-25 minutes or until pears are tender.

5. Remove from the oven, sprinkle with shredded coconut and chopped walnuts.

6. Serve warm.

Nutritional Value:

- Calories: 180

- Healthy Fats: 10g

- Fiber: 8g

- Vitamin K: 10mcg

- Cooking Time: 25 minutes

3. AIP-Friendly Pumpkin Coconut Pudding
Ingredients:

- 1 cup canned pumpkin puree (unsweetened)

- 1/2 cup coconut milk (AIP-friendly)

- 1 tablespoon maple syrup (AIP-friendly)

- 1 teaspoon cinnamon

- 1/2 teaspoon ginger powder

- 1/4 teaspoon nutmeg (optional)

Preparation:

1. In a bowl, whisk together pumpkin puree, coconut milk, maple syrup, cinnamon, ginger powder, and nutmeg.

2. Refrigerate for at least 1 hour to allow flavors to meld.

3. Spoon into serving bowls and garnish with a sprinkle of cinnamon.

Nutritional Value:

- Calories: 150

- Healthy Fats: 10g

- Fiber: 6g

- Vitamin A: 15000IU

- Cooking Time: 5 minutes + chilling time

4. AIP-Friendly Chocolate Avocado Mousse

Ingredients:

- 2 ripe avocados

- 1/4 cup unsweetened cocoa powder

- 1/4 cup coconut milk (AIP-friendly)

- 2 tablespoons maple syrup (AIP-friendly)

- 1 teaspoon vanilla extract (AIP-friendly)

Preparation:

1. In a blender, combine avocados, cocoa powder, coconut milk, maple syrup, and vanilla extract.

2. Blend until smooth and creamy.

3. Refrigerate for at least 1 hour.

4. Spoon into serving cups and enjoy this rich and indulgent mousse.

Nutritional Value:

- Calories: 220

- Healthy Fats: 18g

- Fiber: 8g

- Iron: 2mg

- Cooking Time: 10 minutes + chilling time

5. AIP-Friendly Coconut Vanilla Chia Pudding

Ingredients:

- 1/4 cup chia seeds

- 1 cup coconut milk (AIP-friendly)

- 1 tablespoon honey (AIP-friendly)

- 1 teaspoon vanilla extract (AIP-friendly)

- Fresh berries for topping

Preparation:

1. In a bowl, whisk together chia seeds, coconut milk, honey, and vanilla extract.

2. Refrigerate for at least 4 hours or overnight, stirring occasionally.

3. Spoon into serving bowls and top with fresh berries.

Nutritional Value:

- Calories: 180

- Healthy Fats: 12g

- Fiber: 10g

- Protein: 4g

- Cooking Time: 5 minutes + chilling time

These dessert recipes are tailored to align with the Autoimmune Hepatitis Diet principles. Adjust portion sizes as needed and consult with healthcare professionals for personalized advice. Enjoy these delightful and nourishing treats!

Amidst the challenges of Autoimmune Hepatitis, find solace in your ability to adapt, learn, and grow. You are not defined by your diagnosis; you are defined by your resilience

Chapter 4: Mindful Eating and Lifestyle Changes

Stress Reduction Techniques

In the journey towards managing Autoimmune Hepatitis through a specialized diet, it is crucial to recognize the impact of stress on overall well-being. Stress can play a significant role in triggering or exacerbating autoimmune conditions, including Autoimmune Hepatitis. This section of the cookbook focuses on practical and effective stress reduction techniques that can complement the dietary approach, promoting holistic healing.

1. Mindful Breathing Exercises:

Engaging in mindful breathing exercises can be a powerful tool to alleviate stress. Techniques such as deep diaphragmatic breathing, box breathing, or progressive muscle relaxation help activate the body's relaxation response, reducing the production of stress hormones.

2. Meditation and Mindfulness Practices:

Incorporating meditation and mindfulness practices into daily life can enhance emotional well-being. Simple mindfulness meditation or guided imagery exercises can provide a sense of calm and mental clarity, fostering a positive mindset.

3. Gentle Exercise and Yoga:

Physical activity, especially in the form of gentle exercises and yoga, has been shown to reduce stress and promote a sense of balance. These activities not only improve physical health but also contribute to mental and emotional well-being.

4. Adequate Sleep Hygiene:

Ensuring a good night's sleep is essential for stress management. Establishing a consistent sleep routine, creating a calming bedtime environment, and prioritizing sufficient sleep duration can positively impact stress levels and overall health.

5. Art and Creativity Therapy:

Engaging in creative activities such as art, music, or writing can serve as a therapeutic outlet for stress.

Expressing oneself through creative pursuits provides an avenue for self-discovery and emotional release.

6. Social Support and Connection:

Maintaining strong social connections and seeking support from friends, family, or support groups can significantly alleviate stress. Sharing experiences, concerns, and triumphs with others who understand can create a sense of belonging and emotional support.

7. Time Management and Prioritization:

Effective time management and prioritization of tasks contribute to reducing the feeling of being overwhelmed. Breaking tasks into manageable steps, setting realistic goals, and learning to say no when necessary can help create a more balanced and stress-resilient lifestyle.

In the context of managing autoimmune conditions like Autoimmune Hepatitis, stress reduction is not just a complementary aspect but an integral part of overall wellness. By incorporating these stress reduction techniques into daily life, individuals can create a supportive environment that complements the dietary strategies outlined in the cookbook, fostering a holistic approach to health and healing. It's important to recognize that stress reduction is a personal journey, and individuals may find different techniques more suitable for their unique needs and preferences.

Quality Sleep for Recovery

In the intricate puzzle of managing Autoimmune Hepatitis, the significance of quality sleep cannot be overstated. Adequate and restorative sleep plays a pivotal role in supporting the body's immune system, aiding recovery, and contributing to overall well-being. This section of the cookbook delves into the importance of quality sleep and offers insights into establishing healthy sleep habits for those navigating the Autoimmune Hepatitis Diet.

1. The Role of Sleep in Healing: Quality sleep is a cornerstone of the body's natural healing processes. During sleep, the immune system becomes more active, promoting cellular repair and regeneration. For individuals managing autoimmune conditions, including Autoimmune Hepatitis, prioritizing quality sleep is an essential aspect of the recovery journey.

2. Establishing a Consistent Sleep Schedule:

Creating a consistent sleep schedule involves going to bed and waking up at the same time each day, even on weekends. This helps regulate the body's internal clock, enhancing the quality and duration of sleep. Consistency reinforces the natural circadian rhythm, optimizing the body's functions.

3. Creating a Relaxing Bedtime Routine:

A calming bedtime routine signals to the body that it's time to wind down. Engaging in relaxing activities such as reading a book, practicing gentle stretches, or enjoying a soothing herbal tea can prepare the mind and body for a restful night's sleep.

4. Sleep Environment Optimization:

Crafting an optimal sleep environment contributes to better sleep quality. This involves ensuring a comfortable mattress and pillows, controlling room temperature, and minimizing light and noise disturbances. Creating a tranquil sleep space enhances the likelihood of restorative rest.

5. Limiting Stimulants and Electronics before Bed:

Caffeine and electronic devices can interfere with the body's ability to wind down before bedtime. Limiting the consumption of stimulants in the evening and reducing screen time before sleep can contribute to a more relaxed and restful night.

6. Addressing Sleep Disorders:

For those facing challenges with sleep disorders, seeking professional guidance is crucial. Conditions like insomnia or sleep apnea can significantly impact the quality of sleep. Working with healthcare professionals can help identify and address these concerns, tailoring interventions for better sleep outcomes.

7. Stress Reduction Techniques for Better Sleep:

As discussed in the cookbook's stress reduction section, incorporating stress reduction techniques can positively influence sleep quality. Practices such as mindfulness, meditation, and deep breathing exercises can help calm the mind, paving the way for a more tranquil and restful sleep.

Understanding the interconnectedness of sleep and recovery is fundamental for individuals following the Autoimmune Hepatitis Diet. By prioritizing and optimizing sleep, individuals can harness a powerful ally in their journey towards better health. It's important to note that establishing healthy sleep habits is a gradual process, and individuals may need to experiment with different strategies to find what works best for them. The pursuit of quality sleep is an investment in overall well-being and a key component of the holistic approach to managing Autoimmune Hepatitis.

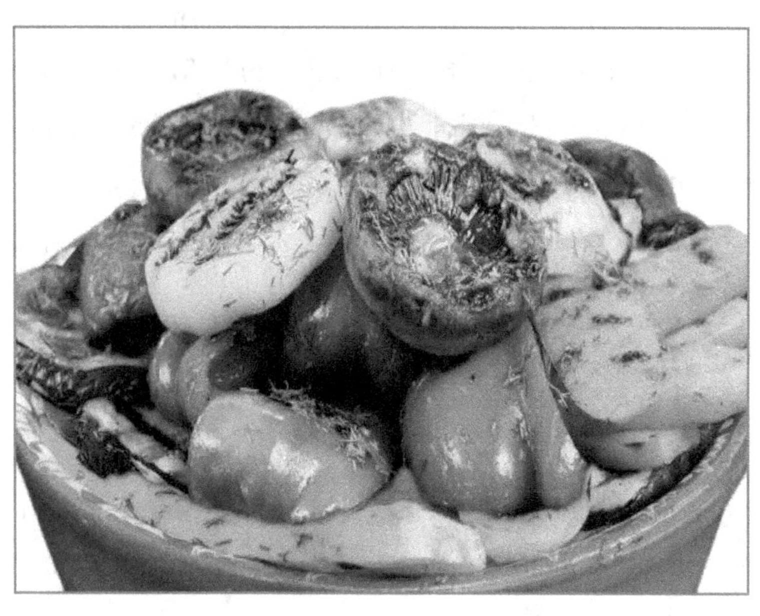

GRILLED VEGETABLES

Chapter 5: Practical Tips and Resources

Grocery Shopping Guide

Navigating the aisles with intentionality is a crucial aspect of successfully implementing the Autoimmune Hepatitis Diet. This Grocery Shopping Guide aims to empower individuals with the knowledge and insights needed to make informed choices when selecting ingredients. By carefully curating your shopping list and being mindful of the foods you bring home, you can create a pantry stocked with items that align with the principles of the Autoimmune Hepatitis Diet.

1. Fresh Produce Section:

- Prioritize organic fruits and vegetables whenever possible.

- Choose a variety of colorful and nutrient-dense options such as leafy greens, berries, sweet potatoes, and cruciferous vegetables.

2. Lean Proteins:

- Opt for lean protein sources such as poultry, fish, and grass-fed or pasture-raised meats.

- Consider including plant-based proteins like legumes and tofu, ensuring they are well-tolerated based on individual dietary needs.

3. Healthy Fats:

- Select heart-healthy fats like avocados, olive oil, and coconut oil.

- Incorporate fatty fish rich in omega-3 fatty acids, such as salmon and mackerel.

4. Gluten-Free Grains:

- Explore gluten-free grains like quinoa, rice, and buckwheat as alternatives to traditional wheat products.

- Check labels for gluten-free certification to ensure adherence to dietary requirements.

5. Nuts and Seeds:

- Include a variety of nuts and seeds, such as almonds, chia seeds, and flaxseeds, for nutrient-packed snacks and meal additions.

- Be mindful of portion sizes due to the potential for high-calorie content.

6. Dairy Alternatives:

- Explore dairy alternatives like almond milk, coconut milk, or hemp milk, taking care to choose those without additives or sweeteners.

- Consider incorporating AIP-friendly options for those following a more restrictive Autoimmune Protocol.

7. Herbs and Spices:

- Enhance flavor without compromising health by incorporating a diverse range of herbs and spices.

- Include anti-inflammatory options like turmeric, ginger, and cilantro for both taste and potential health benefits.

8. Sweeteners:

- Opt for natural sweeteners such as honey or maple syrup, ensuring they meet AIP criteria if necessary.

- Be cautious with artificial sweeteners, which may not align with the diet's principles.

9. Processed and Packaged Foods:

- Minimize processed and packaged foods, as they often contain additives, preservatives, and potential allergens.

- Read labels diligently, avoiding ingredients that may trigger autoimmune responses.

10. Beverages:

- Choose hydrating beverages like water, herbal teas, and coconut water.

- Minimize or eliminate sugary drinks, and exercise caution with caffeinated beverages.

11. Meal Planning Staples:

- Stock up on essentials for meal planning, including broth (preferably homemade), AIP-friendly seasonings, and AIP-approved flours for baking.

12. Label Reading Tips:

- Familiarize yourself with label terminology and look for certifications such as "gluten-free" or "AIP-friendly."

- Be vigilant about potential hidden ingredients or additives that may not align with the Autoimmune Hepatitis Diet.

Arming yourself with knowledge while grocery shopping is a proactive step toward success on the Autoimmune Hepatitis Diet. By selecting wholesome, nutrient-dense foods, you're not only supporting your body's healing process but also savoring a variety of delicious and satisfying meals. Remember, the Grocery Shopping Guide is a dynamic tool that can evolve as you become more attuned to your body's needs and preferences. Happy and mindful shopping!

Dining Out Strategies

Embarking on the Autoimmune Hepatitis Diet doesn't mean sacrificing the joy of dining out. Navigating restaurant menus with mindfulness and planning can empower individuals to savor delicious meals while adhering to the dietary principles. This section provides invaluable strategies for dining out, ensuring that your restaurant experience aligns with the Autoimmune Hepatitis Diet.

1. Research and Choose Wisely:

- Before heading out, research restaurants known for their commitment to fresh, whole ingredients.

- Opt for establishments with customizable menu options, accommodating dietary preferences.

2. Communicate Dietary Needs:

- Don't hesitate to communicate your dietary needs to the server. Ask questions about ingredients and preparation methods to ensure they align with the Autoimmune Hepatitis Diet.

3. Focus on Whole Foods:

- Choose dishes that emphasize whole, unprocessed foods. Grilled proteins, steamed vegetables, and simple salads are often safe and flavorful choices.

4. Avoid Common Triggers:

- Be aware of common triggers like gluten, dairy, and excessive added sugars. Request modifications to exclude these ingredients if necessary.

5. Build Your Plate:

- Many restaurants offer customizable options. Build your plate with lean proteins, a variety of colorful vegetables, and healthy fats like olive oil or avocado.

6. Be Mindful of Sauces and Dressings:

- Sauces and dressings can contain hidden ingredients. Request them on the side or inquire about AIP-friendly alternatives.

7. Inquire about Cooking Methods:

- Ask about the cooking methods used. Grilling, steaming, or baking are often healthier options compared to frying or heavy sautéing.

8. Embrace Ethnic Cuisines:

- Explore ethnic cuisines known for their use of fresh, flavorful ingredients. Mediterranean, Japanese, or Thai cuisines often offer diverse options that align well with the Autoimmune Hepatitis Diet.

9. Plan for Social Situations:

- Inform friends and family about your dietary restrictions when planning social gatherings at restaurants. This helps create a supportive and understanding environment.

10. BYO AIP-Friendly Snacks:

- For times when safe options might be limited, bring AIP-friendly snacks, such as nuts or fresh fruit, to supplement your meal.

11. Scan Menus in Advance:

- Reviewing menus online before arriving can help you make informed choices, reducing stress and ensuring a more enjoyable dining experience.

12. Choose Sides Wisely:

- Sometimes, sides offer the most AIP-friendly options. Mix and match sides to create a satisfying and compliant meal.

13. Stay Hydrated:

- Hydration is essential. Opt for water or herbal teas instead of sugary or caffeinated beverages.

14. Express Gratitude:

- When restaurants accommodate your dietary needs, express gratitude. Positive feedback encourages establishments to continue offering inclusive menu options.

Dining out on the Autoimmune Hepatitis Diet can be a pleasurable experience with thoughtful planning and communication. By following these strategies, you can confidently enjoy restaurant meals while supporting your health and adherence to the Autoimmune Hepatitis Diet. Remember, each dining experience is an opportunity to savor delicious, nourishing food tailored to your specific dietary needs.

In the face of Autoimmune Hepatitis, remember: your strength is a testament to resilience, and your journey is a testament to courage. Keep going, warrior

Chapter 6 Conclusion

Celebrating Progress

As you reach the conclusion of this Autoimmune Hepatitis Diet Cookbook, it's essential to pause and acknowledge the remarkable journey you've undertaken towards better health and well-being. Celebrating progress is not just a recognition of dietary accomplishments but a reflection on the resilience, determination, and self-care that have been integral to your path.

1. Small Wins Matter:

- Celebrate the small victories. Whether it's successfully preparing an AIP-friendly meal or resisting the temptation of non-compliant foods, each achievement contributes to your overall progress.

2. Mindful Reflection:

- Take a moment to reflect on the positive changes you've experienced. Consider how your relationship with food, your body, and your health has evolved since embracing the Autoimmune Hepatitis Diet.

3. Nourishment beyond the Plate:

- Recognize that nourishment goes beyond the plate. The journey you've embarked on encompasses not just dietary choices but a holistic approach to health, encompassing stress reduction, quality sleep, and self-care.

4. Empowerment through Knowledge:

- The knowledge gained throughout this cookbook empowers you to make informed choices about the foods you consume. Understanding the impact of nutrition on autoimmune health positions you as an active participant in your well-being.

5. Culinary Exploration:

- Embrace the joy of culinary exploration. The Autoimmune Hepatitis Diet has likely introduced you to new ingredients, cooking techniques, and flavors. Celebrate the diversity of your palate and the creativity in your kitchen.

6. Gratitude for Support:

- Express gratitude for the support you've received, whether from friends, family, or healthcare professionals. Their encouragement has played a vital role in your journey.

7. Revel in Self-Care:

- Celebrate the self-care practices you've integrated into your routine. Whether it's moments of mindfulness, adequate sleep, or regular exercise, these actions contribute to your overall well-being.

8. Future Wellness Goals:

- As you celebrate progress, consider setting future wellness goals. These goals can be both dietary and lifestyle-oriented, creating a roadmap for continued growth and health.

9. Share Your Journey:

- Share your journey with others who may be on a similar path. Your experiences, challenges, and successes can inspire and support those navigating the complexities of autoimmune health.

10. Embrace Flexibility:

- Recognize that progress is not linear. There may be moments of challenge, and that's okay. Embrace flexibility in your approach, and always prioritize what feels nourishing for both your body and spirit.

In concluding this cookbook, remember that celebrating progress is an ongoing and dynamic process. Your journey is unique, and every step forward is a testament to your dedication to health and vitality. As you continue to explore, learn, and savor the benefits of the Autoimmune Hepatitis Diet, may each celebration be a reaffirmation of your commitment to a life of balance, resilience, and well-deserved joy.

Here's to your health and the exciting chapters that lie ahead!

Living with Autoimmune Hepatitis is a marathon, not a sprint. Pace yourself, celebrate the victories, and remember that your endurance and spirit will carry you through

WEEKLY MEAL PLANNER

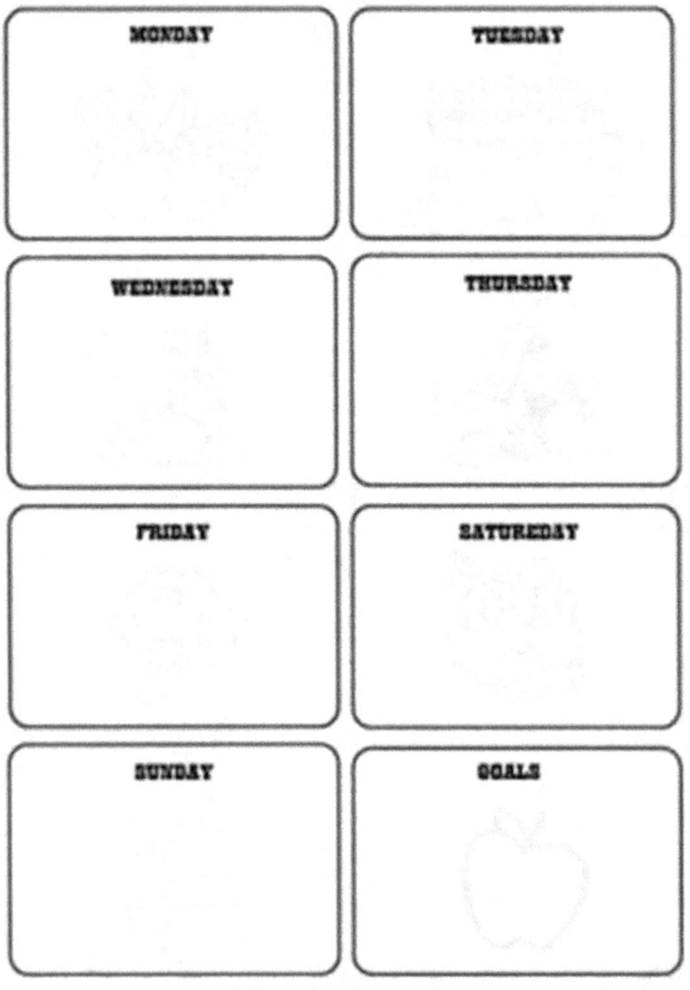

WEEKLY MEAL PLANNER

MONDAY	TUESDAY

WEDNESDAY	THURSDAY

FRIDAY	SATURDAY

SUNDAY	GOALS

WEEKLY MEAL PLANNER

MONDAY	TUESDAY

WEDNESDAY	THURSDAY

FRIDAY	SATURDAY

SUNDAY	GOALS

WEEKLY MEAL PLANNER

MONDAY	TUESDAY

WEDNESDAY	THURSDAY

FRIDAY	SATURDAY

SUNDAY	GOALS

WEEKLY MEAL PLANNER

MONDAY	**TUESDAY**
WEDNESDAY	**THURSDAY**
FRIDAY	**SATURDAY**
SUNDAY	**GOALS**

WEEKLY MEAL PLANNER

MONDAY	TUESDAY
WEDNESDAY	THURSDAY
FRIDAY	SATURDAY
SUNDAY	GOALS

WEEKLY MEAL PLANNER

MONDAY	TUESDAY
WEDNESDAY	**THURSDAY**
FRIDAY	**SATURDAY**
SUNDAY	**GOALS**

WEEKLY MEAL PLANNER

MONDAY	TUESDAY

WEDNESDAY	THURSDAY

FRIDAY	SATURDAY

SUNDAY	GOALS

WEEKLY MEAL PLANNER

MONDAY	TUESDAY

WEDNESDAY	THURSDAY

FRIDAY	SATURDAY

SUNDAY	GOALS

WEEKLY MEAL PLANNER

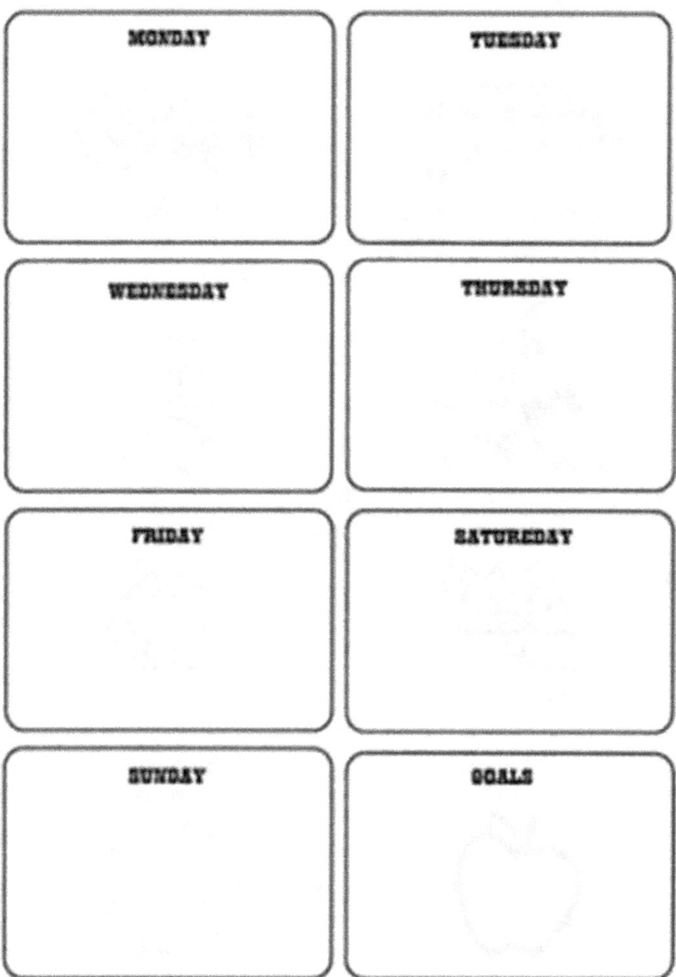